Bubonic Plague: Navigating America's Battle Against Rodent-Borne Diseases

Understanding the Threat, Protecting Your Health, and Building Resilient Communities in the Face of Rodent-Borne Disease

NUEL VICTOR

Table of Content

Chapter 1:

The Black Death Returns: A History of Bubonic Plague

Modern headlines hint at a forgotten terror: Bubonic plague, emblematic of medieval despair, has returned in the 21st century. Understanding the history of this ancient disease is essential to understanding its modern resurgence, despite media hype. The bubonic plague's devastating impact, transmission secrets, and various forms are examined in this chapter.

Imagine a dark world where death stalks the streets and kills quickly. This was the terrifying truth of the Black Death, the worst bubonic plague pandemic ever. This invisible enemy ravaged Europe and Asia in the mid-1300s, killing 50 million people, a third of Europe's population. The vivid descriptions from that time depict swollen lymph nodes, fever-racked bodies, and a chilling darkness over communities. European economic, social, and religious life was forever changed by this ancient scourge, demonstrating its destructive power.

The Unknown Criminal: Yersinia Pestis

What evil force caused this historical pandemic and its modern recurrences? Rodents harbour the deadly bacterium Yersinia pestis. The disease is naturally stored in black rats' blood due to this resilient microorganism. While the black rat is mostly blamed for the Black Death, other rodent species can also carry the bacteria, complicating plague ecology.

Imagine an invisible enemy that could overthrow empires and change history. Yersinia pestis causes bubonic plague, which has plagued humans for millennia. Understanding the resilient microorganism behind the Black Death is crucial to solving past outbreaks and preventing future ones.

Rod-shaped gram-negative bacilli like Yersinia pestis have unique cell walls. Despite its simplicity, this organism has complex weapons. Its fimbriae help it stick to host cells, and its proteins help it avoid the immune system. After entering, Yersinia pestis releases toxins that cause inflammation, tissue damage, and organ failure.

This bacterial villain goes beyond attacking humans. The disease thrives in black rat blood, a natural reservoir. However, Yersinia pestis has multiple hosts. It can manipulate fleas, its insect vector, which is impressive. Fleas become more likely to bite rodents and humans due to the bacterium, perpetuating transmission.

The enemy Yersinia pestis isn't static. It has evolved with its hosts to resist antibiotics and environmental changes over centuries. This adaptability challenges modern medicine, emphasising the need for ongoing research and treatment development.

Scientists are obsessed with Yersinia pestis's every move. Researchers are solving the mystery of this invisible enemy by studying its complex structure and life cycle. Genetic sequencing is revealing how the bacterium evolves and spreads, improving prevention and control.

Unraveling Transmission: Rodent to Human

Preventing outbreaks requires understanding how Yersinia pestis jumps from rodents to humans. Most transmission is through flea bites, tiny parasites that feed on rodent and human blood. When a flea bites a person, bacteria can enter the bloodstream and cause disease. Inhaled respiratory droplets from coughing victims spread pneumonic plague, a rare but deadly disease. Although rare, this form is highly contagious and a public health risk.

A chilling reminder of our vulnerability to microscopic enemies, bubonic plague doesn't magically jump from rats to humans. This chapter unravels the complex transmission chain between Yersinia pestis, its rodent hosts, and unsuspecting humans.

Fleas: Tiny Hitchhikers of Doom

Imagine a bloodthirsty hitchhiker with a deadly cargo in its tiny belly. Fleas are the main vector of Yersinia pestis from rodents to humans. These adaptable parasites bridge the rat and human worlds by feeding on their blood.

When a flea feeds on an infected rat, Yersinia pestis grows in its gut. Interestingly, the bacteria manipulate the flea, preventing digestion and causing starvation and irritability. Desperate fleas bite more, increasing the risk of bacteria transfer to humans.

When infected fleas bite humans, they inject saliva and possibly Yersinia pestis. The immune system usually stops bacteria from establishing itself. If the bacteria overcome these defenses, they enter the body.

Yersinia pestis travels through the lymphatic system. It often starts in the lymph nodes, where immune cells fight bacteria. The bubonic plague's characteristic buboes—swollen, painful lymph nodes—form on this battlefield.

Although fleas are the main carriers, other routes exist. Coughed respiratory droplets spread pneumonic plague, a more dangerous form. High contagiousness makes this form a bigger public health risk. Rarely, direct contact with infected tissue or fluids can spread the disease.

Transmission goes beyond fleas and bites. Recent research suggests additional players. Ticks are being studied as carriers, highlighting the need for ongoing research and vigilance.

Understanding the complex transmission network helps us prevent outbreaks. Flea and rodent control are vital public health efforts. Breaking the transmission chain requires early detection and treatment of infected people.

Humans unknowingly contribute to this complex drama. Poor sanitation encourages rodent breeding, increasing flea exposure. Public education about hygiene and waste disposal reduces the risk.

Understanding transmission paths helps us overcome fear and act. Respecting the invisible forces can help us defend against this ancient enemy and build a healthier future.

Bacterial, Pneumonic, And Septicemic Plague

Bubonic plague was most common during the Black Death and remains so today. Its hallmark is painful lymph node swelling, called buboes, in the groyne, armpit, or neck. The illness is debilitating due to fever, chills, and muscle aches. Yersinia pestis can also be severe:

Pneumonic plague: Rapidly progressing form causing extensive coughing, bloody sputum, and respiratory distress. It is contagious and deadly if untreated.

In septicemic plague, bacteria enter the bloodstream directly, bypassing the lymph nodes. It causes widespread infection, organ failure, and rapid death without treatment.

Knowing plague's different faces helps people and communities spot outbreaks and get medical help.

Understanding the Past, Planning the Future

The bubonic plague's history shows its destructive power. Modern medicine has greatly reduced its mortality rate, but understanding its transmission routes, forms, and historical impact is essential to addressing its current and future challenges. Recognising the past and using informed public health strategies, we can prepare for the resurgence of this ancient disease and ensure a better future for ourselves and future generations.

Chapter 2: Rodent Reservoirs and Urban Sprawl: The Modern Landscape

While the bubonic plague conjures up images of medieval misery, it also has a disturbing contemporary relevance. While medical advancements have lessened its impact, understanding the relationship between Yersinia pestis, its rodent reservoirs, and the changing human landscape is critical for navigating its resurgence. This chapter delves into the hidden world of wild rodents, investigates the impact of urbanization on this delicate balance, and considers the potential role of climate change in altering the plague's geographical spread.

Yersinia pestis does not exist in isolation. It thrives in a complex ecological dance with wild rodents, most notably ground squirrels, prairie dogs, and other burrowing species. These creatures serve as natural reservoirs, transporting bacteria without succumbing to their effects. This delicate balance has existed for millennia, with little effect on human populations.

Urban Sprawl: Disrupting Balance

However, the spread of urban sprawl threatens this harmony. As cities grow, they encroach on these wild areas, fragmenting natural landscapes and displacing rodent populations. These displaced rodents frequently seek refuge in urban outskirts, bringing them into closer contact with humans and their homes. This increased interconnectivity creates ideal conditions for flea-borne transmission, blurring the distinction between wild and urban areas and paving the way for potential outbreaks.

Urban environments unintentionally provide a buffet for hungry rodents. Overflowing garbage cans, unsecured food sources, and insufficient waste management provide sustenance and breeding grounds, resulting in thriving rodent populations. This increase in density heightens the risk of flea infestation and disease transmission.

Beyond Bricks and Mortar: Environmental Change.

The story does not conclude with urban sprawl. Climate change and land use practices are also important factors. Drought and habitat loss can cause wild rodents to migrate, potentially spreading the plague to new areas. Warming temperatures may also make it easier for Yersinia pestis to survive and spread in flea populations, potentially expanding the disease's geographic reach.

Predicting the future impact of these factors is a complex task. Scientists are actively investigating these complex relationships, utilizing ecological modeling and disease mapping to better understand potential outbreak risks. This knowledge allows for the development of targeted public health interventions, focusing on areas with high rodent populations, potential flea infestations, and conducive environmental conditions for plague transmission.

The bubonic plague does not respect national boundaries. Understanding the dynamic relationships that exist across global landscapes is critical for international collaboration and coordinated public health strategies. Sharing information, best practices, and resources on rodent control, early detection, and rapid response is critical for reducing the risks posed by this ancient disease in our modern world.

Rethinking our Relationship with Rodents: Demons or Villains?

Not quite. While rodents may play a role in plague transmission, understanding their importance in ecosystems is critical. Responsible waste management, sustainable land use practices, and community-based rodent control programmes can all help to reduce the risk of conflict and disease transmission while protecting these critical components of our natural world.

By navigating the complex landscape of rodent reservoirs, urbanization, and environmental change, we gain the foresight and tools required to coexist with Yersinia pestis without succumbing to fear or overlooking critical ecological balances. This approach enables us to protect our communities while respecting the interconnectedness of our planet, fostering a future in which the bubonic plague is a historical footnote rather than a looming threat.

Chapter 3:

Recent Outbreaks of Bubonic Plague the US

An unexpected resurgence of the bubonic plague, a disease that was once thought to be a relic of the past, has been observed in the United States in recent years. Cases that have been documented have surfaced in a number of different regions, which shed light on the ongoing danger that rodent-borne diseases pose to contemporary contemporary society.

The specter of the bubonic plague, a disease that is famously associated with the destruction that occurred during the middle ages, may appear to be firmly relegated to the dusty pages of history. Nevertheless, rumors of its revival in recent years serve as a chilling reminder that this long-standing foe has not been defeated; rather, it has been peacefully sleeping for quite some time. The bubonic plague has made an unwelcome comeback, demonstrating its ability to adapt and exploit vulnerabilities in our modern world. This is despite the fact that advances in medicine have significantly reduced the mortality rate associated with the disease. The investigation of these recent outbreaks is not merely an exercise in morbid curiosity; rather, it is an essential step in gaining an understanding of the development of the threat and strengthening our public health defenses. By looking into the shadows of these reappearances, we are able to gain valuable insights that will enable us to better predict, prevent, and contain future outbreaks. This will ensure that the Black Death will continue to be a chapter that has been closed and will not be a harbinger of the future.

Latest Incidents and Their Locations

The resurgence of the bubonic plague has been especially noticeable in the western regions of the United States, which are characterized by environmental conditions that are favorable to the growth of rodent populations. Within the year 2019, for example, there were multiple cases reported in the states of Colorado, California, and New Mexico. The endemic nature of the disease in certain regions was brought into sharp relief by these outbreaks, which served as timely reminders.

Additionally, the demographics that are impacted by these outbreaks are diverse, ranging from rural communities to suburban neighbourhoods. Despite the fact that urban outbreaks have been observed, which presents public health officials with a unique set of challenges, urban outbreaks have traditionally been associated with rural settings.

The following are some of the affected locations:

·   A significant number of cases have been reported in the state of New Mexico, particularly in the more rural areas of the northern region.

·   It has been reported that outbreaks have taken place in the southern regions of the state of Colorado, including regions that have high rodent populations.

·   There have been multiple cases reported in various regions of California, including the southern and northern regions.

·   It has been documented that outbreaks have occurred in the northern regions of the state of Arizona.

· Additionally, there have been cases of bubonic plague reported in the southern regions of the state of Oregon.

· The disease has been reported in the far western regions of Nevada, which is located in the state of Nevada.

Because these areas are considered to be hotspots, which are places where the disease has reemerged, it is imperative that targeted surveillance and control measures be implemented.

Different Factors That Contribute to Outbreaks

The resurgence of the bubonic plague in the United States can be attributed to a number of different factors. The ecological disruption that is caused by urbanization and climate change is a significant factor. This disruption causes the habitats of rodents to be altered, which in turn increases the likelihood that humans will come into contact with infected animals. In addition, the lack of adequate sanitation infrastructure and improper waste management practices create environments that are favorable for the growth of rodent populations, which further exacerbates the risk of disease transmission.

In addition, the expansion of human settlements into regions that were previously devoid of human habitation brings people into closer proximity with rodent reservoirs, which ultimately results in an increased risk of disease transmission. Because marginalised communities frequently lack access to adequate healthcare and pest control services, socioeconomic factors, such as poverty and homelessness, also play a role in amplifying the risk of plague transmission. This is because those communities are more likely to be affected by the plague.

Obstacles to Overcome When Detecting and Diagnosing

In contemporary settings, the detection and diagnosis of the bubonic plague present significant challenges due to the rarity of the disease and the nonspecific symptoms it exhibits. Due to the fact that the initial symptoms of plague, which include fever, chills, and swollen lymph nodes, are similar to those of other common illnesses, it is difficult for medical professionals to effectively identify cases of plague in a timely manner.

As an additional factor that contributes to delays in diagnosis and treatment, the lack of awareness among healthcare professionals regarding the possibility of plague in particular regions is a contributing factor. In addition, the laboratory confirmation of plague necessitates the utilization of specialized testing facilities, which may not be easily accessible in all healthcare settings, thereby further complicating the diagnostic process.

In conclusion, the resurgence of the bubonic plague in the United States highlights the ongoing danger that is posed by diseases that are transmitted by rodents in today's society. In the past few years, there have been documented cases that have brought to light the necessity of increased surveillance, improved sanitation practices, and increased awareness among both healthcare professionals and the general public generally. Addressing the factors that contribute to outbreaks and overcoming the difficulties associated with detection and diagnosis are essential steps that must be taken in order to effectively mitigate the impact that plague has on public health in the United States.

Chapter 4:

Public Health Initiatives: Surveillance, Prevention, and Control

In the United States, public health surveillance systems for plague rely heavily on a coordinated network of federal, state, and local agencies to effectively monitor and respond to outbreaks. These surveillance efforts use a combination of active and passive surveillance techniques to detect and track plague cases in both human and animal populations.

Centre for Disease Control and Prevention (CDC)

The Centres for Disease Control and Prevention (CDC) is the national authority for plague surveillance. The CDC works with state and local health departments to collect and analyse data on reported cases of plague. The agency oversees the National Notifiable Diseases Surveillance System (NNDSS), which requires healthcare providers to report plague cases to their state health departments. The CDC then collects and analyzes this information to identify trends and patterns in disease transmission.

State and Local Health Departments

State and local health departments play an important role in plague surveillance within their respective jurisdictions. They are in charge of investigating suspected cases, conducting laboratory tests, and reporting confirmed cases to the CDC. In addition, state health departments may implement targeted surveillance programmes in high-risk areas or populations to look for signs of plague activity.

Laboratory surveillance

Laboratory surveillance is a critical component of plague surveillance efforts, allowing for early detection and confirmation of cases. Yersinia pestis, the bacterium that causes plague, can be detected in clinical specimens using diagnostic tests like polymerase chain reaction (PCR) assays and culture techniques. Positive laboratory results are communicated to health authorities for further investigation and response.

Wildlife surveillance

Wildlife surveillance is critical for monitoring plague activity in animal reservoirs, particularly among rodent populations. State and federal agencies run surveillance programmes to sample and test wild rodent populations for signs of plague infection. This information aids in identifying areas with a higher risk of human exposure and informing targeted interventions, such as rodent control.

Syndromic Surveillance.

Syndromic surveillance systems use non-specific indicators of illness, such as emergency department visits or school absenteeism rates, to detect outbreaks early. While not limited to the plague, these systems can provide early warning of potential disease clusters or unusual patterns of illness that may warrant further examination.

In summary, the existing public health surveillance systems for plague in the United States take a multifaceted approach, including human case reporting and investigation, laboratory testing, wildlife surveillance, and syndromic surveillance. These systems enable early detection of plague activity, allowing for timely intervention and control measures to reduce the impact on public health.

Strategies to Prevent Plague Outbreaks

To prevent plague outbreaks, a comprehensive approach must be taken that addresses all of the factors that contribute to disease transmission. Rodent control, public education, and community engagement are key strategies for preventing plague outbreaks.

Rodent Control

1. Integrated Pest Management (IPM) uses various methods to control rodent populations, such as habitat modification, exclusion, trapping, and chemical control. IPM is intended to reduce rodent populations while minimizing environmental impact and risk to non-target species.

2. Environmental Management: Improving sanitation and waste management can reduce rodent populations by eliminating their food and shelter sources. Effective rodent control requires proper food and garbage storage, sealing building cracks and openings, and keeping outdoor areas clean.

3. Public health agencies can implement vector control programmes to target high-risk areas or

populations for plague transmission. These programmes may include targeted insecticide applications, rodent baiting, and monitoring of rodent populations for signs of plague activity.

Public Education

1. Public health agencies can use targeted awareness campaigns to educate the public on plague risks and preventive measures. These campaigns may include distributing educational materials, organising community events, and disseminating information through media channels.

2. Educating healthcare providers and the public about plague symptoms can help with early detection and treatment. Raising awareness of plague symptoms such as fever, chills, and swollen lymph nodes can encourage people to seek medical attention right away if they suspect they have been exposed to the disease.

3. Preventive measures: Preventive measures, such as avoiding contact with wild rodents, wearing protective clothing when outdoors in plague-endemic areas, and using insect repellent to avoid flea bites, can all help to reduce the risk of infection.

Community Engagement

1. Community Partnerships: Collaborating with community organizations, leaders, and stakeholders can increase support for plague prevention efforts. Community partnerships can help identify and address specific needs and challenges in affected communities.

2. Community Empowerment and Capacity Building: Providing training, education, and resources can help communities take ownership of plague prevention initiatives, improving resilience and sustainability. Building community capacity to implement rodent control measures, conduct surveillance activities, and respond to outbreaks

can help improve overall preparedness and response efforts.

3. Cultural Sensitivity: Effective community engagement requires understanding and respecting cultural practices and beliefs regarding rodent control and disease prevention. Tailoring outreach efforts to affected communities' cultural norms and preferences can increase receptivity and adherence to preventive measures.

Public health officials can reduce the risk of plague outbreaks while also protecting the health and well-being of vulnerable populations by implementing a combination of rodent control measures, public education campaigns, and community engagement strategies.

Current Prevention And Control Methods Face Challenges And Limitations.

While there are various methods for preventing and controlling plague outbreaks, their effectiveness is hampered by a number of challenges and limitations. Understanding these challenges is critical for developing more effective disease-spread mitigation strategies.

1. Resistance to Rodenticides: Over time, some rodent populations may develop resistance to commonly used rodenticides, making chemical control methods less effective. This resistance can complicate pest management efforts, necessitating the development of alternative control strategies.

2. Environmental Concerns: Chemical rodenticides can harm non-target species and contaminate soil and water. Balancing the need for effective pest control with environmental stewardship poses a significant challenge in plague prevention efforts.

3. Implementing integrated pest management (IPM) strategies requires collaboration among various stakeholders, such as government agencies, pest control professionals, and community members. Coordinating these efforts and ensuring consistent adherence to IPM principles can be

difficult, especially in resource-constrained environments.

4. Limited Healthcare Access: In plague-endemic areas, marginalized communities may face limited access to healthcare services. Limited access to healthcare facilities and diagnostic testing can cause delays in the detection and treatment of plague cases, increasing the risk of transmission and spread.

5. Challenges in Diagnosing Plague: Non-specific symptoms and specialized laboratory testing make diagnosing plague difficult. In areas where plague is uncommon, healthcare providers may lack experience recognising and diagnosing the disease, causing delays in treatment and public health response.

6. Public Perception and Stigma: Plague outbreaks can cause fear and stigma in affected communities, impacting social and economic outcomes. Misinformation and misconceptions about the

disease can exacerbate stigma and impede public health efforts to effectively manage outbreaks.

7. Limited Resources for Surveillance and Control: Public health agencies with limited resources may struggle to allocate resources for plague surveillance, prevention, and control. Limited funding, personnel, and infrastructure can stymie efforts to implement comprehensive prevention and control strategies.

8. Globalization and Travel: Today's interconnected world allows infectious diseases, such as plague, to spread quickly across borders. International travel and trade raises the risk of importing and exporting plague cases, complicating efforts to contain outbreaks and prevent re-emergence in previously unaffected areas.

Addressing these challenges necessitates a multifaceted approach that includes scientific research, community engagement, and policy formulation. Investing in innovative technologies, improving surveillance capabilities, and strengthening healthcare systems can help overcome barriers to effective plague prevention and control, ultimately reducing the disease's impact on affected populations.

Chapter 5:

Medical Response: Treatment and Vaccination

Several antibiotics are effective for treating various types of plague, including bubonic, septicemic, and pneumonic plague. Antibiotic therapy should be started as soon as possible to ensure successful treatment and avoid complications from plague. The antibiotic used is determined by the clinical presentation of the disease as well as the patient's overall health. Antibiotics to treat the Bubonic Plague:

1. Streptomycin.

Streptomycin is the primary treatment for bubonic and septicemic plague. Streptomycin is an aminoglycoside antibiotic that inhibits bacterial protein synthesis and is highly effective against

Yersinia pestis, the bacterium that causes plague. It is typically administered intramuscularly or intravenously, with a treatment duration of 7-10 days.

2. Gentamicin

This is an aminoglycoside antibiotic that effectively treats plague, specifically bubonic and septicemic forms. Administered intramuscularly or intravenously, it works similarly to streptomycin. Gentamicin is a reliable alternative to streptomycin for treating plague infections.

3. Doxycycline

This is a broad-spectrum tetracycline antibiotic used to treat plague, including bubonic, septicemic, and pneumonic forms. It inhibits bacterial protein synthesis and is available in oral and intravenous formulations. Doxycycline is a popular outpatient treatment option that can replace streptomycin or gentamicin.

4. Ciprofloxacin

This is a fluoroquinolone antibiotic used to treat plague infections. It inhibits bacterial DNA synthesis and is available in both oral and intravenous formulations. Ciprofloxacin can be used to treat plague when aminoglycosides and tetracyclines are not available or are contraindicated.

Effectiveness in Different Types of Plague

• Antibiotic therapy is effective in treating bubonic plague, with prompt initiation resulting in a positive outcome in most cases. Streptomycin, gentamicin, doxycycline, and ciprofloxacin are all effective treatments for bubonic plague, and the antibiotic used is determined by the patient's age, underlying health conditions, and the infecting strain's antibiotic susceptibility.

• Septicemic Plague: Yersinia pestis bacteria spread to the bloodstream, causing systemic infection. Antibiotic therapy is critical for treating septicemic plague and avoiding complications like septic shock and disseminated intravascular coagulation (DIC). Streptomycin, gentamicin, doxycycline, and ciprofloxacin are all effective treatments for septicemic plague, and the duration of treatment can be extended to ensure complete bacterial eradication.

• Pneumonic Plague is the most severe and rapidly progressive form of plague, causing respiratory symptoms and high mortality rates if not treated. Antibiotic therapy is essential for treating pneumonic plague and preventing secondary transmission of the disease. Streptomycin, gentamicin, doxycycline, and ciprofloxacin are all effective treatments for pneumonic plague; however, treatment should begin as soon as symptoms appear to maximise effectiveness.

In summary, streptomycin, gentamicin, doxycycline, and ciprofloxacin are among the antibiotics available for treating various forms of plague. Prompt antibiotic therapy initiation is critical for successful treatment and prevention of plague complications, and the antibiotic used is determined by factors such as the clinical presentation of the disease, the infecting strain's antibiotic susceptibility, and patient-specific factors.

Bubonic Plague Vaccine Development and Its Potential Use in Outbreak Control.

Plague vaccine development has been an ongoing research area for decades, but there is currently no widely available vaccine for human use. However, several vaccine candidates have shown promise in preclinical and early-stage clinical trials, raising the prospect of developing an effective plague vaccine. This is the Current State of Plague Vaccine Development:

1. Recombinant Protein Vaccines: Using Yersinia pestis antigens to stimulate an immune response is one approach to developing a plague vaccine. These vaccines typically target specific proteins involved in the pathogenesis of plague, such as the F1 and V antigens. Preclinical research has demonstrated that recombinant protein vaccines can induce protective immunity against plague in animal models.

2. Live Attenuated Vaccines: These vaccines contain weakened strains of the Yersinia pestis bacterium, which can still trigger an immune response. These vaccines mimic natural infections and can cause long-term immunity. Several live-attenuated vaccine candidates have been developed and tested in animal models, yielding promising efficacy and safety data.

3. Subunit Vaccines: Purified components of the Yersinia pestis bacterium, like outer membrane proteins or polysaccharides, can trigger an immune response. Subunit vaccines provide greater safety

than live attenuated vaccines while still protecting against plague. Several subunit vaccine candidates have been tested in preclinical studies and shown efficacy in animal models.

4. DNA Vaccines: These vaccines introduce plague antigens into host cells, causing an immune response. DNA vaccines have the potential for rapid development and production while eliciting both humoral and cellular immune responses. While DNA vaccines for plague show promise in preclinical studies, more research is needed to determine their efficacy in humans.

Potential Role In Outbreak Control.

The development of a safe and effective plague vaccine could have a significant impact on outbreak control and prevention efforts, especially in high-risk populations or plague-endemic areas. A vaccine could help to reduce disease spread by immunizing susceptible individuals and protecting them from both natural infection and potential bioterrorism threats involving Yersinia pestis.

In the event of a plague outbreak, vaccination could be used as a preventative measure to keep the disease from spreading among at-risk populations like healthcare workers, first responders, and people living in plague-endemic areas. Vaccination could also be used as part of a larger public health response strategy, alongside other control measures like surveillance, case detection, and antibiotic treatment.

Furthermore, a plague vaccine may have broader implications for global health security, aiding in the mitigation of emerging infectious diseases and bioterrorism threats. Public health officials can improve their preparedness and resilience to this potentially devastating disease by investing in research and development efforts to advance plague vaccine candidates. However, more research is required to overcome the remaining challenges and obstacles to vaccine development, ultimately bringing a safe and effective plague vaccine to market.

Future Advances In Diagnostics, Therapeutics, And Prophylaxis.

Future advances in plague diagnostics, therapeutics, and prophylaxis have the potential to completely transform our ability to prevent, detect, and treat this lethal disease. Here are some possible advancements in each of these fields:

Diagnostics:

1. Rapid diagnostic tests can detect Yersinia pestis antigens or genetic material directly from patient samples, allowing for timely plague diagnosis in resource-limited settings or during outbreaks.

2. Advances in biosensors and nanotechnology may enable highly sensitive and specific diagnostic tools for detecting plague biomarkers in patient samples, requiring minimal equipment and expertise.

3. Whole genome sequencing can identify virulence factors, antibiotic resistance genes, and transmission patterns in Yersinia pestis strains, guiding outbreak investigations and treatment decisions.

4. Machine learning and AI techniques can analyze large clinical datasets.

Therapeutics:

1. Novel antibiotics with improved efficacy, safety, and resistance profiles could offer alternative treatment options for plague, especially in cases of drug-resistant strains or intolerance to current antibiotics.

2. Immunomodulatory Therapies: Enhancing the immune response to Yersinia pestis infection may complement antibiotic treatment and improve patient outcomes by reducing systemic inflammation and tissue damage.

3. Bacteriophage Therapy: Bacteriophages, viruses that infect and kill bacteria, have potential as an alternative or adjunctive treatment for plague infections. Phage therapy may provide targeted and specific treatment options, particularly for drug-resistant strains of Yersinia pestis.

4. Host-Targeted Therapies: Targeting immune signaling pathways or host cell receptors may offer new ways to combat plague and lower mortality rates.

Prophylaxis:

1. Developing safe and effective plague vaccines is a top priority for public health authorities. Future vaccine candidates may use novel antigen formulations, adjuvants, or delivery systems to improve immunogenicity and efficacy.

Passive immunization with monoclonal antibodies or convalescent plasma containing anti-plague antibodies may offer temporary protection against infection in high-risk individuals, such as healthcare workers or military personnel.

3. Chemoprophylaxis: Pre-exposure prophylaxis with antibiotics or antiviral agents can protect individuals at risk of plague exposure, such as laboratory workers or travelers visiting plague-endemic areas. This reduces the likelihood of infection from Yersinia pestis.

4. Vector Control: New insecticides, traps, and genetic modification can reduce the spread of plague-carrying fleas and rodents, lowering the risk of human transmission.

By leveraging future advances in diagnostics, therapeutics, and prophylaxis, public health officials can improve our ability to prevent, detect, and treat plague infections, ultimately lowering the disease's impact on affected populations. Continued investment in research and development efforts is required to turn these promising advances into practical tools and strategies for combating plague in the coming years.

Chapter 6:

Beyond Bubonic Plague: Other Rodent-Borne Diseases

In addition to plague, there are several serious rodent-borne diseases that endanger public health in the United States. Two notable cases are hantavirus pulmonary syndrome (HPS) and leptospirosis.

1. Hantaviral Pulmonary Syndrome (HPS):

HPS is a severe respiratory illness caused by hantavirus infection in rodents, specifically deer mice in the United States. HPS is transmitted to humans through inhaling aerosolized virus particles from rodent urine, droppings, or saliva in enclosed spaces like cabins, barns, or outbuildings. Symptoms include fever, muscle aches, fatigue, and cough, which can quickly progress to severe respiratory distress and pulmonary edoema, resulting in respiratory failure and death in up to 38% of cases.

HPS is rare but can cause sporadic outbreaks, especially in rural areas with high rodent populations. Rodent control measures, avoidance of contact with rodent-infested areas, and proper ventilation of enclosed spaces are all effective prevention strategies.

2. Leptospirosis is a zoonotic disease caused by pathogenic strains of Leptospira bacteria shed in the urine of infected rodents and animals. Humans can contract leptospirosis through contact with contaminated water, soil, or food, or through skin or mucous membrane breaks in contact with infected animal tissues or fluids.

Symptoms range from mild flu-like illness to severe manifestations such as jaundice, kidney failure, and pulmonary haemorrhages. Severe cases can be fatal if not treated.

Leptospirosis is more common in tropical and

subtropical regions, but can also occur in temperate climates, especially after heavy rainfall or flooding. Prevention measures include avoiding contact with potentially contaminated water or soil, wearing protective clothing and footwear in high-risk environments, and implementing rodent control measures to reduce the risk of transmission from rodents to humans.

Both hantavirus pulmonary syndrome and leptospirosis emphasise the importance of understanding and mitigating the risks associated with rodent-borne diseases, such as implementing effective rodent control measures, practicing good hygiene, and raising awareness among healthcare providers and the general public about the diseases' signs, symptoms, and prevention strategies.

The possibility of future outbreaks necessitates comprehensive preparation.
Future outbreaks of rodent-borne diseases, such as plague, hantavirus pulmonary syndrome (HPS),

and leptospirosis, remain a major concern due to a variety of factors, including environmental change, urbanization, and globalization. Comprehensive preparedness efforts are required to reduce the impact of these outbreaks and safeguard public health. Here's an analysis of the potential for future outbreaks and the importance of comprehensive preparedness.

1. Environmental Factors: Climate change, habitat destruction, and ecosystem alterations can all have an impact on rodent populations and their interactions with humans, raising the risk of disease transmission. Climate change, in particular, may cause shifts in the geographic distribution of vector-borne diseases like plague and HPS, increasing the risk of outbreaks.

2. Urbanization and encroachment: Humans' proximity to rodent reservoirs increases the risk of disease transmission. Poor sanitation, overcrowded living conditions, and insufficient waste management practices in cities can foster rodent infestations and disease outbreaks.

3. Globalization and Travel: International travel and trade accelerate the spread of infectious diseases, such as rodent-borne diseases, across borders. Travelers visiting endemic areas may unintentionally spread infections to new areas, resulting in localized outbreaks or the introduction of novel pathogens to vulnerable populations.

4. Antimicrobial Resistance: The emergence of antimicrobial-resistant bacteria, such as Yersinia pestis, presents a significant challenge for treating rodent-borne diseases. Drug-resistant pathogens may reduce antibiotic efficacy while increasing the severity and duration of outbreaks, emphasizing the need for alternative treatment strategies and resistant strain surveillance.

5. Limited Public Health Infrastructure: Inadequate public health infrastructure, especially in resource-limited settings, can hinder rodent-borne disease surveillance, diagnosis, and response. A lack of laboratory capacity, healthcare resources, and trained personnel may cause delays in detection and containment, allowing outbreaks

to spread.

Comprehensive preparedness efforts are required to address these issues and reduce the impact of future rodent-borne disease outbreaks. To ensure timely intervention and containment, key preparedness components include surveillance and early detection of rodent populations, disease prevalence, and outbreaks.

• Public Health Education: Educating healthcare providers, first responders, and the public about rodent-borne diseases, preventive measures, and early detection and treatment can reduce transmission and severity of outbreaks.

• Integrated pest management strategies can prevent diseases like plague and HPS by controlling rodent populations, reducing vector habitat, and limiting human exposure to infected animals.

• Strengthening public health infrastructure, such as laboratories, healthcare systems, and emergency response, is crucial for managing outbreaks and providing timely medical care to affected individuals.

• Investing in research to develop diagnostics, therapeutics, and vaccines for rodent-borne diseases can improve prevention, diagnosis, and treatment, reducing morbidity and mortality during outbreaks.

To summarize, the possibility of future outbreaks of rodent-borne diseases emphasizes the importance of comprehensive public health preparedness measures. By addressing environmental, social, and healthcare challenges, as well as implementing proactive measures to detect, prevent, and control outbreaks, we can reduce the impact of these diseases and protect the well-being of vulnerable populations.

Conclusion:

Beyond Bubonic Plague - Building a Resilient Future

Recent plague outbreaks have taught public health officials valuable lessons and highlighted the ongoing threat posed by this ancient disease. Here are key takeaways from recent outbreaks and potential future threats:

Lessons learned:

1. Vigilance/surveillance: The significance of ongoing surveillance and vigilance against plague cannot be overstated. Recent outbreaks have highlighted the importance of robust surveillance systems for detecting plague activity and facilitating early detection and response efforts.

2. Prompt and coordinated response efforts are crucial for containing plague outbreaks and preventing spread. Effective communication, collaboration among local, state, and federal agencies, and rapid resource deployment are critical to reducing disease spread.

3. Community Engagement and Education: Providing accurate information about plague risks, preventive measures, and treatment options builds trust and cooperation during outbreaks. Public health education should be culturally sensitive and tailored to the needs of diverse populations.

4. One Health Approach: Plague is a zoonotic disease, which means it can spread from animals to people. Adopting a One Health approach that considers human, animal, and environmental health is critical for comprehending and mitigating the complex factors influencing plague transmission.

5. Antimicrobial Resistance: Antimicrobial-resistant strains of Yersinia pestis present a significant challenge in treating plague infections. To address this threat, antimicrobial resistance needs to be monitored and alternative treatment strategies developed.

Potential future threats:

1. Climate change can impact the distribution and abundance of rodent populations, affecting the geographic spread of plague transmission. Changes in temperature and precipitation patterns may create new ecological conditions favorable to plague outbreaks in previously unaffected areas.

2. Globalization and Travel: International travel and trade increase the risk of importing and exporting plague cases, which can spread the disease across borders. Tourism, migration, and commerce may inadvertently introduce plague to new areas or reintroduce it to previously eradicated regions.

3. Urbanization and Encroachment: Humans' proximity to rodent reservoirs leads to increased disease transmission risk. Urban slums and informal settlements with inadequate sanitation infrastructure are especially vulnerable to plague outbreaks.

4. Conflict, displacement, and humanitarian crises can disrupt public health infrastructure, hinder response efforts, and promote disease transmission. Conflict-affected populations may be more vulnerable to plague due to overcrowding, malnutrition, and a lack of access to medical care.

5. Biological Warfare and Bioterrorism: Plague has historically been used as a biological weapon, and the intentional release of Yersinia pestis by malicious actors is a concern. Surveillance for suspicious activities, response plan development, and collaboration with law enforcement and national security agencies should all be part of the preparedness efforts.

In conclusion, recent plague outbreaks have highlighted the ongoing threat posed by this ancient disease, emphasizing the importance of preparedness, surveillance, and collaboration in mitigating its impact. Public health officials can work to prevent and control plague outbreaks while also protecting the health and well-being of vulnerable populations by learning from previous experiences and addressing potential future threats.

How to Take Responsibility for Your Personal Health and Community Well-Being Against the Bubonic Plague.

Empowering people to take responsibility for their own health and community well-being is critical for building resilience, fostering a prevention culture, and improving overall public health outcomes. Here are a few ways to empower people in this regard:

1.   Health Education and Awareness:

• Provide culturally sensitive and accessible health education materials to help individuals make informed health decisions.

• Educate people on common health risks, preventive measures, and the significance of early disease detection and treatment.

• Provide resources and support to enhance individuals' health literacy and understanding of medical information.

2.   Promote Healthy Habits:

• Encourage regular exercise, balanced nutrition, adequate sleep, and stress management.

• Promote preventive health measures like vaccinations, screenings, and regular check-ups.

• Provide support and resources for quitting smoking, preventing substance abuse, and promoting mental health.

3.   Community Engagement and Support:

• Create a sense of belonging through social networks, neighborhood associations, and community organizations.

• Encourage participation in community initiatives, volunteer activities, and public health campaigns to enhance community well-being.

• Offer platforms for individuals to share their experiences, knowledge, and resources with their community.

4.   Empowerment through Knowledge and Skills:

• Empower individuals to advocate for their health needs and navigate the healthcare system efficiently.

• Provide training programmes and workshops on first aid, CPR, and emergency preparedness.

• Encourage leadership development and advocacy for health equity and social justice in communities.

5. Access to Resources and Support Services:

• Ensure equal access to healthcare services, preventive screenings, and treatment options for all community members.

• Help individuals access support services like counseling, mental health resources, and social assistance programmes to improve their overall well-being.

• Encourage policies and initiatives that address social determinants of health, including poverty, housing instability, and food insecurity, to promote healthier communities.

By empowering people to take an active role in managing their health and contributing to community well-being, we can foster a health culture that promotes resilience, equity, and better public health outcomes. We can create healthier, more resilient communities for all by taking collective action and empowering individuals.

www.ingramcontent.com/pod-product-compliance
Lightning Source LLC
Chambersburg PA
CBHW060210260726
48658CB00005BA/1967